Becoming Vegan:

The Key to Going Green, Losing Weight and Having a Happier and Healthier Life.

Table of contents

Introduction

I want to thank you and congratulate you for downloading the book, "Becoming Vegan Today: The Key to Going Green, Losing Weight and Having a Happier and Healthier Life."

This book contains proven steps and strategies on how to start being vegan today, lose weight the vegan way and live a healthy happy life. The book begins by exploring the different types of vegans to help you make an informed decision of the type of vegan you would like to be. The following chapters outline what vegans eat and how to lose weight and achieve the body size that you desire. The next chapter describes how the vegan diet will make you healthy by preventing the development of a number of health conditions. Finally, the book outlines the challenges that may befall you as a vegan and how to overcome them. By the time you turn to the last page of this book, you will have a clear idea of how to become a vegan and live a healthy, happy, and long life!

Thank you again for downloading this book. I hope you enjoy it!

Chapter 1

What is a vegan?

If you are planning to become a vegan, you should first know that there are different types of vegans and choose the best option that fits you. In general, vegans exclude all animal-derived food from their meals. You will not find meat, eggs and dairy products on the vegans' food list. A vegan will also avoid processed food, some wines and even refined sugar. Are you an animal lover? If so, you might want to be an ethical vegan rather than a dietary vegan. While a dietary vegan primarily avoids eating animal-derived food, an ethical vegan not only avoids consuming food derived from animals, but also products that researchers have used in experiments conducted on animals as well as using animals in activities such as bull fighting or carrying of luggage.

By being a vegan, you will do the following:

- Eat food derived from plants only
- Wear clothes made from other materials other than wool, leather and silk.
- Use household products and cosmetics that are not animal-tested
- Withdraw support of the use of animals as a source of labor

Vegan versus Vegetarian

Don't be confused, a vegan is not similar to a vegetarian. You should stay focused in your quest to becoming a vegan by first highlighting the differences between a vegan and a vegetarian. It not only helps you when make food choices, but also in knowing what challenges to expect in your new life as a vegan. Vegetarians only exclude certain animal products from their diet and will still consume some animal-based products. Vegans, on the other hand, avoid not only consumption, but also any possible use of animals and products derived from them. It, therefore, means that you have to get rid of your silk, woolen and leather outfits as well as animals such as donkeys and oxen that you might be using as a source of labor.

Chapter 2

What to eat, the Vegan Diet

Despite the vegan diet being primarily plant-based, it contains all the nutrients that the body needs for proper functioning. The good thing is that if you do become a vegan, you will have completely eradicated cholesterol from your diet. In addition, you will be consuming food that is low in saturated fats and calories and high in fiber, cancer-fighting antioxidants, as well as complex carbohydrates.

The primary nutrients that every individual should provide his or her body with are proteins, carbohydrates, vitamins, fats and micronutrients. A vegan diet also includes magnesium, potassium, folate, vitamin E, anti-cancer photochemicals as well as enzyme boosters and co-workers of antioxidants. If you have been taking many animal products, you might be worried of the repercussions of going vegan. Worry no more, this chapter gives you a detailed outline of what to eat in order to meet the requirements of your body.

Proteins

The number one plant-based product that should appear on your food list is the soybean. It not only contains proteins, but also amino acids that are essential for your body. Essential amino acids are a type of amino acids that your body cannot process. For this reason, you must supply them to the body through the food that you consume. In addition, all types of beans and peas are an excellent source of proteins. You should take plenty of chicken peas, seeds, broccoli, mushrooms, lentils, whole-wheat bread, oatmeal and walnuts to obtain sufficient proteins.

Iron

Your body requires iron for the development of strong muscles. Meat contains a lot of iron. Now that you will not be consuming meat, you have to consume plant-based food that contains large quantities of iron. You will have to take green leafy vegetables in almost every meal. Spinach is the best source of Iron. The best thing about consuming spinach is that it will also supply you with Vitamin C, a vitamin that assists your body to absorb iron. You should also eat lentils, beans, black-eyed peas, nuts, oatmeal, sunflower seed, nutritional yeast and quinoa. All these contain iron.

Omega-3s

Omega-3s supply your body with fatty acids that contribute to the healthy functioning of the heart, brain, skin and joints. However, the primary source of omega-3s is the fish. Fish have cholesterol and toxins that are harmful to the body. Vegans do not consume fish. For this reason, you should get your omega-3s from seaweeds such as algae. Remember that fish get their share of omega-3s from seaweeds too. In addition to algae, consume canola oil, flaxseeds and walnuts.

Calcium

The primary sources of calcium for vegans are beans, broccoli, kale, collard greens, almonds and sesame tahini. You should also drink rice milk and lots of orange juice. Vegans do not eat meat but do take pseudo meats. These products mimic meat in appearance and textures. You should consider tofu as it would provide your body with as much calcium as meat would.

Vitamin D

Vitamin D is a vitamin that your body can synthesize on exposure to the sunlight. What happens if you do not get exposure to sunlight? It does not mean that you will not get Vitamin D; you can obtain Vitamin D from milks derived from plants as well as orange juice.

Vitamin B12

You should take vitamin B12 supplements and multivitamins in order to supply your body with sufficient amounts of the nutrient. Look for soy, rice milk and nutritional yeast fortified with Vitamin B12 when shopping. Cereals and tofu will also provide your body with Vitamin B12.

Chapter 3

Do it, Go Vegan!

You can become a vegan by three main steps depending on your situation.

1.Substitution method

By this method, you only substitute non-vegan food with vegan food. Although you will easily find substitutes for meat and dairy products, you should not expect them to have a similar texture and taste as meat and dairy products. However, the substitutes will supply your body with the same nutrients as meat and dairy products would.

Substitute baked chicken served with rice and broccoli with a vegan chicken such as a high quality Gardein and Beyond meat brand. Instead of cooking your rice in butter, cook it in vegetable oil or vegan butter such as Earth Balance.

If you love burgers, chose vegan burgers such as the Boca, Gardenburger, Sunshine Burgers and Amy's. The good thing is that you can also make your version of a vegan burger at the comfort of your home. The substitution method is an easier way of beginning a vegan lifestyle. However, you should do away with the meat substitutes if your aim is to lose weight. You should not be keen on the taste of the substitutes you take but concentrate on the fact that you are making the transition to another diet. It will enable you to remain committed to a vegan diet and eat what you are supposed to be eating regardless of taste and flavor.

If you are an expert cook, you might realize that it is easier to adopt a vegan lifestyle by following vegan recipes. You should, therefore, look for recipes as well as follow meat plans but replace the meat with meat analogues derived from soy and gluten.

If you are worried about satisfying hunger, you will be surprised to realize that a vegan meal lacking animal product is as satisfying as a meal with animal products. If you are good at cooking, you will be able to make vegan food that is very similar to non-vegan food.

When cooking, focus on real foods such as those containing whole grains, beans, legumes, vegetables, fruits, seeds and nuts. In fact, you should ensure that you have a balanced diet. You should try different recipes every day to ensure that you do not end up with the same food on your table repeatedly.

3. Learn how to cook

Being vegan is difficult if you do not know how to cook. Firstly, you will have to take almost all your meals at home. Secondly, you might be the only person in your household who lives the vegan lifestyle. Only a few restaurants have vegan foods on the menu. It means that if you do not have a cook in your house, you will have to cook. The need to learn how to cook is inevitable once you become a vegan.

So, how do you learn how to cook?

You can either learn to cook by watching others cook and then doing what you saw them doing when cooking. Do not shy away from making mistakes; we only learn through mistakes. By watching others cook, you not only learn how to cook vegan food but also develop other ideas and techniques that may develop into new recipes. The more you watch others cook, the more you become better at the kitchen.

Alternatively, you can enroll for free cooking classes. You could search for individuals in your community who offer cooking lessons for vegan meals.

Chapter 4

No starving, No fad diets; Lose weight the Vegan Way.

By adopting a vegan diet, you can quickly lose excess weight by following eight tips outlined below.

1.Do not consume junk food.

Although most vegan foods do not contain cholesterol, it does not follow that it cannot make you gain weight. You should keep off from vegan junk food such as organic frozen pizza, which contains soy pepperoni and non-dairy cheese. Also avoid packed vegan food and always ensure that you consume food that cannot rot. If you must take these types of food, do so as sparingly as possible.

2.Familiarize yourself with the shopping market nearby.

By becoming vegan, you commit yourself to taking real food. You should always shop for vegetables and fruits in plenty. Know which parts of the market to find fresh vegetables and fruits. It will save you a lot of time as well as keep you away from food that may tempt you to stop being a vegan. If you are looking forward to losing weight, do not buy synthetic food or otherwise, food that your granny would not recognize as food. By doing so, you will curb yourself from accidental consumption of non-vegan food that could prevent you from losing weight.

3. Other than the grocery shop, expand your 'shopping area' to the farmers' market.

Although groceries may provide a wide variety of farm produce, you are never sure to obtain the best quality products at reasonable prices. In the farmers' market, you are sure to find fresh—straight from the garden—farm produce. The other advantage with shopping from the farmers' markets is that the prices are reasonable. Shopping from these markets is also a way of showing support to the local economy and of reducing the amount of carbon that you release to the atmosphere. In the event that there is no farmers' market in your locality, you can always join a cooperative that can deliver fresh produce to your residence.

4. Flavor your food with herbs and natural seasonings

In order to extract flavor from the vegan foods, vegetable oil or fat is the primary product used in cooking. However, too much of the vegetable oil or fat will hinder your achievement in weight loss. For this reason, use natural herbs and seasonings to bring out the flavor that you desire. The real thing with herbs and natural seasonings is that they are so many, and you can even use a different herb every day of the week to prevent boredom.

5. Shop for organic food

Organic food is food grown in a natural state environment—
organic food producers do not use any chemical in cultivation of
the plants. Organic food contains many nutrients naturally
derived from the soils on which they grew. You will enjoy the
natural flavor of organic food, and your body will derive all the
necessary nutrients from the food. For this reason, you will be
satisfied after a meal and are less likely to overeat or eat snacks
between meals. The result is a healthy weight loss.

6. Eat, eat and eat Oatmeal as often as you can.

Oatmeal will give you sufficient energy that lasts. You should eat oatmeal at breakfast to ensure that you have the energy to see you through the day. For you to gain maximum benefits from an oatmeal breakfast, take it together with apples, bananas, cinnamon, maple syrup, carob powder, maple syrup, flaxseeds, raisins and many other different fruits. Oatmeal not only helps you to lose excess weight but also reduces cholesterol, protects your heart and inherently contains subtle amounts of gluten.

7. Exercise

The best way to lose weight is through exercise and watching what you eat. In fact, experts claim that weight loss is through 80 percent diet and 20 percent movement. You do not have to go to the gym in order to engage in the activity that expends energy. You do not have to run many miles too. All that you have to do is get up and get moving. You should engage in an activity that you love such as swimming, dancing or even yoga. You could even engage in simple by physical activities such as gardening.

Chapter 5

Go Vegan, Be Healthy!

You will live a healthy and happier life by eating a vegan diet. Your body will develop resistance to the following common health conditions.

Aging

Are you aging faster than your age mates are? The vegan diet will help you remain youthful and full of energy. By being vegan, you will consume a lot of vegetables and fruits that will enable your body to maintain muscle and hence age gracefully. In addition, you will keep your sight even in old age, as cataracts will not appear in your eyes.

Cancer

Researchers have established that a vegan diet can stop the progression of prostate cancer. The vegan diet enables the body to reverse prostate cancer in men diagnosed with the condition. If it can reverse cancer, will it not prevent it? You should eat whole grain, vegetables and variety of fruits to protect yourself from colon cancer. If you are a woman, you will have lesser chances of developing breast cancer than your counterparts who consume dairy products on a regular basis.

Arthritis

Experts advise patients suffering from rheumatoid arthritis to avoid consumption of gluten-loaded products. It alleviates the condition, the patient experiences relief, and lives a near normal life. If you remain a vegan, you will, therefore, escape from developing arthritis and thus live a healthy, pain-free life.

Heart diseases, Hypertension and Diabetes

Scientific research has proven that a vegan diet reduces the probability of developing heart diseases, as well as Type 2 diabetes. If you have Type 2 diabetes, a vegan diet will be appropriate in the event that you are unable to stick to the standard diet prescribed for diabetic patients. A vegan diet does not contain the bad cholesterol that is responsible for cardiovascular diseases and even stroke. Bad cholesterol makes your arteries thin and causes high blood pressure. For this reason, the vegan diet will ensure that your arteries are of the standard dimensions and hence you will not develop hypertension.

Physical Fitness

The vegan diet will enable you to achieve the body weight you have always desired. It will enable you to maintain your correct body mass index (BMI). The good thing is that you will not only be fit but also be energetic to do all the activities you desire to do.

In addition, the vegan diet will help you overcome the problem of bad breath. Bad breath may be a frustrating condition that may prevent you from socializing as you please. With a vegan diet, the bad breath will go, and you can once again begin to socialize, talk with friends and even laugh aloud with confidence. In general, you will be able to enjoy a more fulfilling life as your body odor will improve too. Your hair and nails will be healthy and your self-esteem will go up. The other good thing about being vegan is that you will forget the pain and the inconveniences of allergies.

Osteoporosis

Osteoporosis is a condition characterized by the thinning of bones. You should not be scared of developing the condition if you stick to a vegan diet. A vegan diet is rich in proteins and potassium and contains little sodium and sufficient calcium. In other words, the vegan diet contains these nutrients in a balance that prevents the progressive thinning of bones.

Chapter 6

Watch out!

The vegan diet is effective in achieving a healthy body weight as well as prevention of lifestyle diseases. However, it can cause other health conditions that may make you lead a sad life and even die prematurely. Below are situations that may arise from unbalanced vegan diet and how to prevent you from developing the conditions.

Iron deficiency

Iron is a nutrient that is in plenty in meat. Your source of iron is plant based if you are vegan. Unfortunately, your body does not absorb iron from plants as fast as it absorbs iron from meat. In addition, phytates and fiber oxalates hinder absorption of iron by the body. Impaired absorption of iron thus predisposes you to development of anemia. To ensure your body gets enough iron, consume many leafy green vegetables, beans, lentils, black-eyed peas, oatmeal, sunflower seeds, quinoa and nutritional yeast.

Iodine deficiency

Vegans miss iodine in their diets because most manufacturers extract iodine from animal products. Inadequate iodine predisposes you to a health condition referred to as goiter. In order to gain adequate iodine, you should consume sea vegetables as often as possible.

Vitamin deficiency

As a vegan, you are most likely to develop Vitamin D and Vitamin B12 deficiencies. If you are introducing the vegan diet to your children, be warned that lack of Vitamin B leads to neurodegenerative disorder, neurological disorder and even anemia in children. Deficiency of Vitamin D on the other hand hinders absorption of Phosphorous, which leads to rickets in children. Thus, always ensure that you have an exposure to sunlight for at least 30 minutes if possible and take Vitamin D supplements. Consume Vitamin D fortified drinks and lots of orange juice too.

Malnutrition

If you extend the vegan diet to infants, you should be very keen because death due to malnutrition frequently occurs in children raised on a vegan diet. Always ensure that your infant eats a balanced diet and breastfeed frequently.

Underweight infants

For women, be keen if you are expectant; you might end up delivering an underweight baby if you do not stick to a balanced diet. In order to ensure that you have sufficient nutrients for you and the baby you are carrying, consume nutrient supplements of all the essential nutrients such as calcium, zinc and the vitamins.

Deficiency in Omega-3s

Since most of the omega-3s are present in fish, vegans have a high probability of developing deficiency of omega-3s because they do not eat fish. Deficiency in omega-3s leads to cardiovascular, cancer and even arthritis. In order to gain sufficient omega-3s from your diet, include seaweed in your meals as often as possible. Omega-3s are also in plenty in nuts and seeds such as flaxseeds and walnuts. In case you do not have easy access to this kind of food, please consume omega-3s supplements.

Conclusion

Thank you again for downloading this book!

I hope this book was able to help you to start the vegan diet in the most convenient way.

The next step is to follow the newly adopted diet and lose that extra weight to enjoy a healthy, happy and long life.

Finally, if you enjoyed this book, then I'd like to ask you for a favor, would you be kind enough to leave a review for this book on Amazon? It will be highly appreciated!

www.ingramcontent.com/pod-product-compliance
Lightning Source LLC
Chambersburg PA
CBHW062032280526
45787CB00005B/2290